Thru the Fire

By: Kinyatal Jones

Dedication: To my sons Dj and Man I love you all with everything in me. Thank you for always pushing me to become better.

This book is dedicated to the little girl with no voice.

Prelude:

Job 42:5 NLT, "I had only heard about you before, but now I have seen you with my own eyes."

There was no other man like Job. God bragged on him to the devil. It wasn't until Job entered into his trial where he developed a personal relationship with God. We can serve God and not have that intimate relationship with him. This book is my personal experience of how I found God. Travel with me as we enter the water, river, and fire.

The water: When you pass through the water, I will be with you

As I look into the mirror, the person looking back at me had eyes that hid the pain of abuse, rape, and depression. Her smile holds the joy that was taught by endurance. Legs strengthen from walking the journey alone. Back pain from the weight of the world. Head raised because no matter what she would not allow her circumstances change her posture.

Feet holds her victory. Mouth holds her praise. Hands her surrender. Clothes smells like smoke. Face radiant from being in God's presence.

How can you enter fire but come out unharmed?

Easy, you didn't go through it alone. Sometimes, I wonder how I could endure so much in 31 years. Then I remembered God will not put more on you than you can bear. At 31, I finally realized who I am, not just in God's eyes but as a woman. It took a while to get to this place. Let's start from the beginning.

A person's identity is the fact of being whom or what that person is. As we travel through life our identity is shaped by our experiences and the people we meet.

Kinyatal Sintrel Jones AKA Kydd was born October 25, 1984. Kydd loved to play basketball, run track, read Babysitter Club Books, write poetry, sing, and dance. Music was her love, but dance was her passion. As, a child Kydd never fit in. She was the oldest of three and the product of a teenage pregnancy. She didn't know her biological father.

Who was she? Her father was a high school picture her grandmother gave her. At times her dad seemed like a figment of her imagination. Maybe one day I will meet my biological father. Does she have any other brothers or sisters she thought? Kydd always felt something was missing.

Kydd lived with her grandparents until she was 12. Her Nana was such an angel. She loved Kydd and kept her in church. Kydd's grandfather Papa was her heart. He was the strongest person she knew. He was dealing with kidney disease and diabetes, but he always smiled. He taught her life lessons like "be a woman of your word and to always try to help people whether they deserved it or not."

Kydd started finding her identity outside of her family. In the fifth grade, Kydd met Payne, she was a beautiful girl. She wore fitted pants and cut off shirts. They were inseparable. Kydd was no ugly duckling.

She was caramel in completion, slim, and athletic built. Kydd had a beautiful smile and very outgoing. The interaction with Payne made Kydd want to dress more like her beautiful friend. This was a turning point in Kydd's life because this was the first time, she tried to change who she was to fit the mold of man. When we see what we think is pleasing to man/people we sometimes try to fit into that imagine.

Kydd knew at a young age she did not fit and was not supposed to. The more she tried to the more damage she did to herself. Throughout junior high, Kydd met friends, mainly because she was a class clown. Kydd had a smart mouth and developed a habit of hurting others on purpose. She would cuss you out so bad you would have wished she would have hit you. Kydd felt that if she was funny and good at sports people would be her friend. Kydd wasn't a horrible person she just wanted to hurt you before you hurt you.

The phrase hurting people hurt people was true in her life. If you were laughing with her you couldn't possibly dislike her or hurt, her. At the end of junior high, Kydd met a boy.

Quiet Stream

Duece was her first. He was a thug (well he wanted to be) he really wasn't that cute, but he desired her and that was enough. Duece was the first guy she ever really interacted with. It was a normal day, in middle school Kydd's mother checked her out of school.

The day before Papa was taken to Birmingham because he had gotten sick. Papa told Kydd to be a big girl and take care of the family. It was weird because he usually did not say anything but see you later Pumpkin.

When they arrived at the hospital Nana met them in the waiting room and told Ma and Kydd that Papa just died. Kydd was crushed. If Papa was gone who was gonna love her? The death of Papa was another critical event for Kydd. When we associate who we are with a person and that person leaves so does our identity. This can cause us to look for approval or our identity in others and that is what Kydd did.

One night, Deuce and Kydd was hanging out and he said, "Let's have sex." She didn't know anything about sex. Papa was dead and she just wanted to be loved. So, if he is my first, we will be together forever. After about 5 mins the sex was over and Kydd felt numb, but Deuce looked at her and said love you. But did he?

Deuce was the first of many guys in the pages of Kydd's life.

SILENT TEARS

Awaken from a deep sleep Being Beat I
don't know why I can't bring myself to cry
Wondering why

Silent Screams and Wet tears fill my years
of life

It can't be Gotta be better than this Numbing
the pain with sex Because he claims he loves
me He loves me not Not knowing the seeds
planted in me I want to be free but The mask
has me in bondage

Hello God

Can you hear me?

Darkness n clouds fill my day I pray and
pray No one hears the

Little black skinny girl

Left with the loneliness

Of silent screams n wet tear

The River: Through the rivers, they will not overwhelm you.

All her life not knowing her biological father affected her negatively. The enemy told her that she didn't know because she wasn't worth it. It was the biggest lie the enemy used to keep her in bondage. Throughout the next few years, it was guy after guy numbing the pain for the rejection Kydd experience from her biological father.

High school wasn't all bad. Kydd was a great runner. She was an All Star, All Bi-City, and Wendy's Heissman nominee. Kydd future consisted of track at Florida State. That was until she met Brown Eyes. Brown Eyes was a year older than Kydd. She

12

would skip school and practice to be with Brown Eyes.

Sex was normal for her now. Around Christmas, Kydd started to gain weight and was feeling herself. She loved Brown Eyes but he said she wasn't ready for a relationship. So, Kydd started talking to QB. QB was a star all-around athlete at the rival of Kydd's high school. Heading to work one evening she felt something wasn't right. She went and got a pregnancy test. She took it at work and the results were?

 Her gift was born Aug 30, 2003. The gift almost didn't make it. When Kydd found out she was pregnant her high school coach told her he would pay for an abortion. She thought about the abortion. Her life was over. She wouldn't be able to go to school with a baby. Kydd had slept with QB and

Brown Eyes the same weekend so she was not sure who Jonathan's dad was. She was ashamed because she was now needing Maury's help about finding out who was Jonathan's father.

Kydd didn't want to be pregnant and then the blood came. I can't be bleeding I'm pregnant. The emergency room nurse said you might be experiencing miscarriage. No, Lord you can't let me lose my baby I love him. Lord please let him live. Kydd didn't know what the sex of the baby was but she knew he had purpose. Jonathan was one of the best things that ever happened to her.

College was normal for Kydd. She worked two jobs at times to get extra money for her and Jonathan. Guys continued to be the bandage she used to cope. At 21, Kydd started being serious about God. She started dancing and noticed she had a gift.

Now, Kydd had been dancing in church since she was 12. Now at 21, she was being taught the word and fundamentals of worship.

On fire for God, Kydd still searched for love in the form of a man, a cute one with nice arms to be exact. One day Kydd received a call from a guy she met at a gas station. He asked if he could come over and of course that was cool. They had been talking for a while.

He came over they watched ICEAGE and Jonathan went to sleep. He started kissing on Kydd. Kydd thought wow he is really into me. He started tugging at Kydd's shorts. Kydd stated, "Oh I don't want to have sex." He placed his finger inside her and stated, "You are wet. Yes, you do." Kydd yell, "No I don't get off me." He said, "Man stop you gonna wake up the baby." Kydd laid there and tried to enjoy it. It was really her fault she allowed a stranger to come over.

This experience brought her to God. She decided I'm going to just take care of Jonathan and serve. The next couple years, Kydd grew in ministry. She was getting invitations to dance all over the city. She was graduating college and things were looking good for her now. Her son was happy and healthy. She was growing in God. Then she met Best Friend.

Can They See

Screams Tears Growing fears I walk around, and no one hears The moans inside I try to hide I did my best I dress the part Then why is my life torn apart But lord you said Your blood you shed For me to have everlasting life you paid the price So why don't I feel the joy you claim is real Why are they ignoring me? **Can they not see?**

It is killing me Behind the makeup I hide the clothes so perfect They fit my shape It makes them say she has it all together I jump, I praise, I call out your name **but they cannot see**

The hurt in me I'm trying to be Who you called me to be Through the guilt and the shame The insults and the pain Your glory I still claim They never will see me because you hide me in the shadows They will only see a glimpse Your love covers the scars Hides the pain and Your love rains and reigns So now I know I am not to be seen just echoes of the wind Gentle breezes that kisses on the cheek

That encourages me that my place in the world is not more worthy than a squirrel That even if they never see A child a God I will always be.

The Fire: When you walk through the fire, you will not be burned or scorched, nor will the flame kindle upon you

Best Friend was younger than Kydd but he captured her heart. He made her believe in love again. He loved her son as his own and her unconditionally. After a yearlong engagement, Kydd and Best Friend were married. Shortly after came the birth Keith. The two were happy and in love. The first 2 years were great.

In 2013, God called her into ministry. Kydd always knew she was different. During a worship conference a prophet gave a name to Kydd's gift. He called her a prophet. Everything made sense to Kydd now.

She knew things without knowing the people or their situation, when she danced it changed the atmosphere, and why she declared the impossible. At that moment, Kydd told God I will walk with you forever and surrendered her life to God. She was a true servant her life was fruitful her ministry was growing. Then suddenly....

"Jonathan is having a seizure, Ma screamed through the phone." Kydd was so scared no devil you can't have him he's mine she thought. When Kydd arrived at Ma's house Jonathan was having what appeared to be a seizure. They rushed him to the emergency room and there they stated the lack of oxygen caused the seizure like spells. Kydd felt relieved it wouldn't happen again, BUT it did.

The entire Memorial Day weekend Jonathan continued to have these spells. They were getting worse. Kydd had taken him to every local emergency room and now they were being advised to take him to Birmingham. The doctors at Children's Hospital told Kydd that

Jonathan was having pseudo seizures. It was happening because Jonathan was under a lot of stress.

How can a 10-year-old be that stressed?

Jonathan started sharing things with Kydd. He was saying some deep-rooted stuff concerning his Brown Eyes (biological dad) and Best friend her husband. Kydd was distraught. How can I love a man that has hurt my son so bad? She asked. He is the only person who will want me, Kydd thought. Kydd prayed and talked with Jonathan she decided to stay with her husband they can get through anything together.

"If she comes here, I'm leaving! Kydd screamed." Kydd was so hurt how can Best Friend even bring up the thought of allowing another woman to move into their home. Kydd packed her and the boys' stuff and left. Best Friend allowed his Female Friend and her children to move into Kydd's home. A home they shared so many good times in. Kydd almost lost her mind. She cried out to God, "Why did you allow this?"

After staying with her parents for a month and a lot of praying the Lord told Kydd to go back home and fight for her marriage. I am crazy for going back Lord why I gotta go back. She was going to counseling. She was stressed at work and home. The doctor placed her on medical leave twice due to stress during this time.

God made her study Hosea. At the time, Kydd did not know why God require her to study the ultimate love story for his people.

Instead she thought, "How can God ask this Hosea to love a hoe? Why is God asking me to love Best friend and he got this woman in my house?

Better yet, Lord why I can't beat her down? Love them? God you are tripping, Kydd thought."

EVENTUALLY, Best Friend female friend left but the damage was done. Kydd asked Best Friend if he wanted to go to counseling. Best Friend stated he was not going to counseling. Kydd fasted and prayed. Lord fix my marriage.

One day, Kydd was crying on the bedroom floor Best Friend came in and looked at her then walked back out. How could he see me in pain and leave the room? Kydd had enough she asked Best Friend to leave. During this time, Kydd thought things would get back on track after some time apart. She was wrong the day Best Friend left was the last day they shared as a couple.

October 2014 Kinyatal turned 30. She had used all her money to move into her own place. She felt horrible. "If I died today, I would be in heaven, Kydd thought." Kydd would not kill herself because she did not want to go to hell. She would often think of suicide because she felt as if what she was living was closed to hell.

Kydd couldn't understand how God could allow her marriage to fail. She did everything God had asked. She danced, taught, prophesied, gave her tithes, and served with everything she was.

Why was this happening? She decided to continue going to church but she was just going to use their Wi-Fi. She had stop wanting to live. She was heartbroken and wondered why God allowed this to happen to her. Even though she was broken hearted she continued to minister in dance whenever she received an invitation. She did not want to live but if she did, she would praise God.

She felt as if she was sinking deeper into despair. One day, her friend Red Shirt called, Red Shirt told Kydd that God wasn't going to help her fight for something that wasn't meant to be kept. Red shirt also told her God was not going to keep allowing her to play. If she died, she would not be in God's grace. Kydd repented that day and started back on the right track.

Life After the Storm

This is my testimony this is my life. When I decided to finally put it all on paper, I wanted to sugarcoat it. God told me I had to be transparent in telling it. The beauty of my testimony is I am here to share it. The things that I shared were not to hurt my family or my ex-husband.

It was to give a voice to little girls and young women who do not know their identity. I declare that the uncertainty of who you are ends today. If you are reading this book know that there is purpose in your process. God allowed you to turn the pages because of this very moment.

God wants you to know your identity in him. In the beginning of Isaiah 43: 2 it talks about the waters. Water composes over 50 percent of our body. That means that without the right amount of water our bodies cannot function correctly.

John 4:14 "But those who drink the water I give will never be thirsty again. It becomes a fresh, bubbling spring within them, giving them eternal life." Jesus in numerous places in the bible spoke on him being water. Why? This is to show that a relationship with him is vital.

 Just like you should drink 8 gallons of natural water daily the same should be with your relationship with Christ. God wants you to know who you are in him. The water I faced in life was trying to find my identity. Just like in the natural body not knowing who you are can stop the growth of becoming your true self.

Have you ever wondered why a situation did not take you out? Did you ask God why did this person leave? These questions create our identity. If you do not know your value, you will not walk in the fullness of who you are in God.

When you pass through the waters, I will be with you; this part of the scripture indicates that as you find your identity God will be with you. You will pass through the trial in victory. You will not die. God ensures us that we will go through the trial/water. So, shout for victory now because you will make it.

Through the rivers, they will not overwhelm you the water or my lack of knowledge of who I had caused me to build up bad behavior. I did not know who I was in Christ, so I became who others wanted me to be. I became a whore, class clown, etc. just to gain temporary identity. As you can see when you do this the buildup of water can cause a river or a steady flow of pain. I used my biological father not being there as a crutch. My legs could not get strong because I was constantly hopping on that crutch.

In order to find out who you are in Christ you must look at yourself and see what in your life represents the water. Majority of your identity is focused around what? What issue overwhelms you? Be real with yourself. I did not notice I had an issue with men until I was separated. I started trying to get over the pain of what I was going through by jumping into bed with another issue or person.

One thing I realized is I turned back into 15-year-old Kydd. Every time something resembled the rejection, I received from my dad I acted like a 15-year-old girl. This happened for 15 years. It was only until someone told me and educated me on why I acted the way I did I understood.

The river is a place where all resolved memories and emotions reside. It is time to now address the water damage and eliminate the river. The river did not overwhelm me or drown me in that place I went through it.

When you walk through the fire you will not be burned or scorched nor will the flame kindle upon you. When we think of fire we think of a hot miserable place. The fire in my life was the end of my marriage.

Now, I am not a bitter black woman. My ex-husband is a great man he is just not the man for me. True enough he hurt me but that is not the focus of the book. The fire is the trial that caused me to lose my place in God, my peace, and my hope.

For you it may be a rape, divorce, or loss of a loved one. Any reason that can knock you down to the point of not wanting to get up is your fire process. The fire is when you do not think you will live through the trial. The thing about me is I could handle trial.

My endurance level for trouble was high. As, a child I went through a lot, so it was not strange to pray and seek God. When I started being a worshipper, I danced my way out of every storm.

This is where I gain my strength. I was told by so many people I did not know you were going through that or girl you look good for enduring that.

That was God's grace keeping me. Although, I endured the fire I wasn't burn. Now, I do smell like smoke. The fragrance of what I been through is on me and it is my anointing.

I do not identify myself in the things I endured. I find my identity in God. I am unashamed of my testimony because those things caused me to know God in a way, I never knew him before. God became my everything.

When you're doped up on anxiety medicine and all you can do is pray you find strength. My faith muscles were strengthened. Kydd is not a little girl rather than a dynamic strong black woman. She empowers others by unmasking the scars of her heart. I want to encourage you to take the bandage off your wound.

God can not heal you until you rip off the bandage and air it out. Not saying tell your business to everyone but find a trusted person and start talking. Do not be in bondage by family secrets, shame, or wounds of the heart. You are not meant to carry that baggage. It's time for you to become free!

I kept asking God how he wanted me to end this book. I wanted to say something powerful to push you into your freedom. This morning I am emotional. I have been through a lot. I poured my heart into this book. I am being transparent because so many times we walk around like nothing is wrong.

We go to work, take care of kids and family, but we are so broken inside. I walked around for years broken. I realized about 3 months ago that being broken is sometimes the best way to be.

For oil to flow, the container must be turned upside down, broken, or the top must be repositioned. It is the same for you for you to be who God intended you must endure the process of change.

The process may seem to break you, turn life upside down, or reposition you. But know you will make it out the process and really see Beauty of Ashes.

DECLARATION:

I speak to the broken woman. The woman who feels worthless. The woman who must take care of her kids alone, so you do not have time to process the pain. The woman who identity is tied into a man. The woman who keeps the secret of abuse, and rape. The woman who every morning gets up and pretends everything is ok.

Today I declare that woman (your name) will become whole. God died so that you could be free. Yes, things happened throughout your life that may have made you feel that you were in bondage. Today that ends!

Woman you have endured and now are broken. Life has you in position for God and only him to move. He has been moving throughout this book. You identified with a lot of the things I endured. You said a lot of the things I said.

My life is an example of how God can take trial and make beauty. If you see me today, I am worshipping God. The things that happened abuse, rape, teenage pregnancy, and divorce did not take me out. I am not saying it did not hurt. Sometimes I wanted to die. I asked God numerous times to just allow me to die. The great thing about God is he would always give me a way of escape. I could have been ashamed that I been on anxiety medication, raped, divorced, and abused. I could have hidden the fact that at 30 I do not know who my biological father. I am not ashamed.

Everything I endured was for God's glory. It was for this time. So, know that God loves you. He loves you enough to allow me to go through the water, river, and fire to minister to you. You are victorious! You will make it! You are beautiful! God will and can still use you! More than anything remembers no matter what you go through God is there and he will keep his word!

About Author

Kinyatal Sintrel Jones is a mother of 2 boys Demarre' (Dj) and Brandon Jr

(Man). Her boys are her biggest accomplishment. Kinyatal graduated from Columbus State University with a Bachelor of Science in 2008 and Master of Administration in 2013. In 2012, Kinyatal founded Thru the Fire Ministry. A year later, Kinyatal started teaching dance to youth. In 2015, Kinyatal expanded her teaching gifts and is now a Worship Arts Instructor. Kinyatal teaches lyrical, drama, and worship instruments.

In 2020, Kinyatal opened her worship Arts Academy in Phenix City, AL. Her academy is steadily grown as she has students from different churches and nationalities that she teaches how to worship. Kinyatal has written 5 books: Thru the Fire 2016, Angel in the Room 2016, Dancing in the rain 2017, Biblical Expression (2017), and A Walk Thru the Fire creative expression workbook 2019.

Kinyatal is not limited to written expression. She has produced and directed three plays Consuming Fire, Burden Down (2017) and Tis the Season 2019. She also produced and directed her first movie Man in the Mirror (2018) and This Can't B3 Life web series (2019). Kinyatal has one goal, one purpose, one pursuit that is to make God famous in all she does.